IIFYM & Flexible Dieting

**The Ultimate Beginner's "If It Fits Your Macros"
Flexible Macros Calorie Counting Diet Guide -
Everything You Need To Know To Eat All The Foods
You Love and STILL Lose Weight**

By Logan Thomas

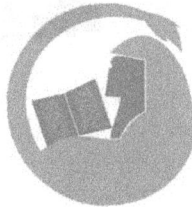

EFFINGO
Publishing

For more great books, visit:
EffingoPublishing.com

Download another book for Free

We want to thank you for purchasing this book and offer you another book (just as long and valuable as this book), "Health & Fitness Mistakes You Don't Know You're Making," completely free.

Visit the link below to signup and receive it:

www.effingopublishing.com/gift

In this book, we will break down the most common health & fitness mistakes, you are probably committing right now, and will reveal how you can quickly get in the best shape of your life!

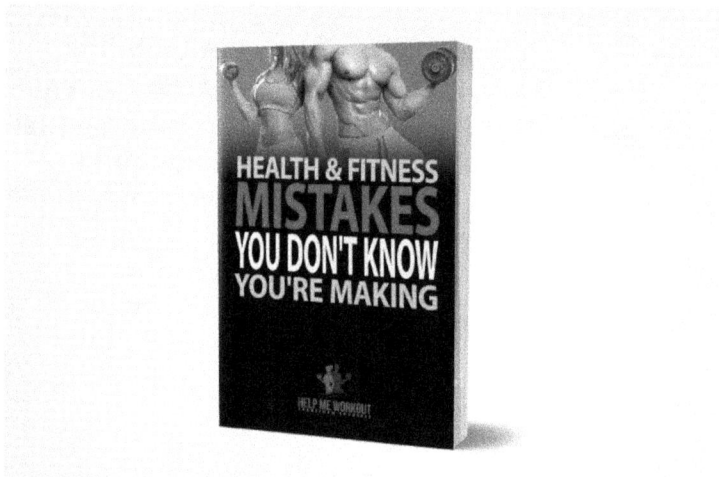

In addition to this valuable gift, you will also have an opportunity to get our new books for free, enter giveaways, and receive other useful emails from us. Again, visit the link to sign up:

www.effingopublishing.com/gift

TABLE OF CONTENTS

INTRODUCTION

Having a healthy body is one of the biggest and most important things you can have. If the body is healthy, it means that you can do whatever you love for much longer. The best way to keep the body healthy is by making sure that the food you eat is healthy. Avoiding junk foods and vices will keep you and your body healthy. Combine those with regular exercise, and you will be in top shape.

But the thing is, not everyone has that option.

Exercising regularly is easier said than done. Not everyone has the time to squeeze exercise in with their busy schedules. It doesn't help that; most of the time, people are too tired to do more physical work when they get home. Another factor can also be laziness or lack of desire to exercise.

So the other option to have a healthy body is to eat healthily. There are a lot of dieting regimes out there right now. But they all have one thing in common: They are ways of controlling what you eat.

In this book, we will be looking at one of these diet regimes or techniques. We hope that by the time you finish reading this, you will be informed about the method. We also hope that you will be able to use the information in this book to become healthier and maintain this life style.

Also, before you get started, I recommend you joining our email newsletter to receive updates on any upcoming new book releases or promotions. You can sign-up for free, and as a bonus, you will receive a gift. Our "Health & Fitness Mistakes You Don't Know You're Making" book! This book has been written to demystify, expose the top do's and don'ts and to finally equip you with the information you need to get in the best shape of your life. Due to the overwhelming amount of misinformation and lies told by magazines and self-proclaimed "gurus," it's becoming harder and harder to get reliable information to get in shape. As opposed to having to go through dozens of biased, unreliable, and untrustworthy sources to get your health & fitness information. Everything you need to help you has been broken down in this book for you to easily follow and to immediately get results to achieve your desired fitness goals in the shortest amount of time.

Once again, to join our free email newsletter and to receive a free copy of this valuable book, please visit the link and signup now: www.effingopublishing.com/gift.

IIFYM: What is it?

Of the many diets out there, they all have one thing in common: They restrict what you eat. For most diets, you can't eat sweets or fatty foods—which is great as too much sugar or fat is bad for you anyway. Others limit your consumption of carbohydrates.

There is a regime that is more flexible. It lets you eat whatever you want—with certain conditions. It is called the IIFYM diet.

The Basics Of IIFYM

IIFYM is an acronym for the phrase "If It Fits Your Macros." It is a dietary regime that helps you lose weight without restricting what you eat. You can eat anything as long as "it fits your macros." We will be discussing more what macros are later in the book. For now, let us just focus on what flexible dieting and IIFYM are.

What you have to understand is that IIFYM does not restrict your diet. You can eat anything you want. To understand IIFYM much more, let us now look into how it works.

How Does IIFYM Work?

IIFYM, or flexible diet, does not control what you eat. You can eat whatever you want. Whether that's pizza, ice cream, cake, or anything you can think of. How does it do this?

Well, first, let us think about what makes the body fat? Your first instinct might be to answer: fatty foods, junk foods, sugar, etc. But, here's the thing—they are not the main reason why you get fat. Sure, they can contribute to it, but they are not the main reasons. This is one of the biggest misconceptions about dieting in general. There is no scientific study which proves that certain foods make you fat. (Feinman & Fine, (2004). What makes you fat is excess calories. These excess calories create a surplus of calories in the body.

IIFYM, generally speaking, lets you control your calorie intake based on the macronutrients. You can eat anything you want as long as it is within limits set by the macros. So, IIFYM is different from other diets. Most diets control what you eat, while IIFYM controls how much. In essence, it is the simplest way to diet. If you want to reduce weight, you just have to lessen the amount of food you eat. But that is an extreme oversimplification. Just drastically reducing your food intake may be harmful instead of helpful. IIFYM is a controlled and calculated way of directing how much you can eat every day.

Later, we will go into much more detail about how you can follow the diet. Be warned—it involves a bit of mathematics.

What Are The Benefits Of IIFYM?

Now that we've discussed what IIFYM is let us now look into the benefits you can get from IIFYM.

You Can Get Your Desired Weight

The biggest and most noticeable benefit of IIFYM is, of course, it helps you control your weight. Weight loss is possible because the calorie and macronutrient intake is reduced by 15-25% if you are following the diet for it. There are also some suggestions that high-protein diets, like IIFYM, increase metabolism, which makes regular weight reduction possible. If you want to gain weight, just increasing the intake of calories and protein will help you gain weight.

It Is Flexible

IIFYM is more than just a diet—It is a litestyle. Because of this, it is much easier to sustain than most diets. Most diets restrict what you eat, which limits what kinds of food you can eat. This leads to you eating just bland or boring foods. Imagine just eating chicken and broccoli every single day. Wouldn't that be boring? With IIFYM, this won't be a problem. This is because the diet is extremely flexible. You can eat anything as long as you keep your calorie intake at the proper amount. Sustaining the diet feels much easier because you are eating a variety of food.

No More "Forbidden" Foods

In IIFYM, you can eat anything. That is the main selling point of this diet. No food is forbidden. Are you craving curry? Go ahead and order one. Do you want fries, a cheeseburger, and a milkshake? Be my guest. As long as you keep in mind your macros and calorie count, you will still be in the clear. This not only makes it easier to stick to the plan, but it allows you to enjoy the process. Most dieting methods are very restrictive, which takes away from most of their benefits. But with IIFYM, what you need most is discipline.

Requires Less Exercise

Because IIFYM reduces the intake of calories, it does not require that much exercise. This is because, when the calculations for macros are done, physical activities are taken into account. This means that even if you have minimal physical activities, you can still follow the diet, and you will still be able to enjoy the effects. This does not mean, of course, that you don't need to exercise. We recommend that you couple the diet with regular exercise to achieve the best results.

Are There Any Drawbacks To The IIFYM?

Now that we have discussed the benefits of IIFYM let us now look into some of its less desirable traits or effects. Just like anything, there are specific cons or drawbacks to the process.

It Is Still A Diet

No matter how flexible the IIFYM diet is, it is still a diet. Just like every other diet out there, there is a consensus that they just don't work in the long run. A lot of people who begin the diet may just stop one day and going back to the way they were before. This often negates some of the progress the diet has made. So to avoid this drawback, it is best to keep yourself motivated while following the diet. As said before, discipline will be your best tool to help you keep up with it. Also, it is much better if you integrate IIFYM into your lifestyle for you to enjoy the benefits much longer. You may also consult with a diet or nutrition professional to tailor fit the diet for you and your needs.

Does Not Care About Micronutrients

The IIFYM diet focuses all of its attention on the macronutrients that you get. It is even in the name of the diet. As such, it does not care at all about the micronutrients like vitamins and minerals. So much time is devoted to tracking the macros and the calorie intake that these micronutrients are ignored. There has been researching that shows the adverse effects of not getting enough micronutrients into the body. The deficiency of micronutrients may even lead to illness. To combat this drawback, make sure that you are taking micronutrients into account. That is one saving grace that the IIFYM diet has: it is flexible. Because of this, you can introduce foods that are part of your meal plan but also contain vitamins and minerals. If this is not possible, you may take multivitamin supplements.

Health Conditions Are Not Accounted For

Not everyone can follow the IIFYM diet. This category includes those who have certain health conditions or those who require special diets. Those with diabetes will have to look out for their intake of carbohydrates, for example. It is possible to tailor the IIFYM diet to still work with certain conditions. Seek help from nutrition professionals or dieticians to find out how to adjust the diet for your medical needs.

Risk Of Eating Disorders

Keeping track of your macronutrients can help you reach your health goals. But that is not the case for every person who wants to try the IIFYM diet. There may be cases when it can trigger disordered eating. Tracking food and fitness can lead to the development of certain eating disorders. Young women are more vulnerable to this scenario. A study shows that 73% of college students who have been diagnosed with eating disorders think that tracking their food, fitness, and other aspects of their nutrition led to or at least contributed to, the development of their disorder. Again, it is essential that you seek a professional opinion from nutrition and healthcare experts before beginning the diet. This is to make sure that you don't have eating disorders, or if you do have them, how to make sure that it will not lead to making your condition worse.

FUNDAMENTALS OF NUTRITION:

CALORIES AND MACROS

The human body has been compared multiple times to a machine. And, to be honest, it somewhat is a machine. It has multiple parts that work together. It has much more value with all the parts together than if they were separated. And if you remove key parts, it will cease to function properly. But the similarities don't end there. Like a machine, the body also needs fuel. The fuel for machines come from multiple things. It can be gasoline, diesel, coal, wind, etc. But the fuel for the human body comes from one basic thing: the food we eat.

Now, what would happen if you put the wrong kind of fuel in a machine? One of three things will happen. One: The machine will not work. This is because the fuel type is incompatible with the machine. For the second scenario, the machine will function but at reduced efficiency. It will not work to its maximum potential. Or worse, in the third scenario, the machine will be destroyed.

Something similar may end up happening to the body. As we said, the body needs fuel. And that fuel comes from the food we eat. But if the wrong kind of fuel inside the body, it will either stop functioning, function at a reduced rate, or something may be damaged. For example, what would happen to your body if you eat something you are allergic to? The body will react a certain way.

Another example is the consumption of alcohol. The body does not need alcohol to function properly. Alcohol impedes normal body functions. So what happens when you consume too much alcohol? You will get drunk. Your senses will be dulled, and the body will, essentially, stop functioning properly—at least until the effects wear out. That is the main difference between a machine and the human body. A machine does not have a way to self-repair while the human body does. Over time, some damage may be reversed or repaired.

But the best and most effective way to keep the body running smoothly and functioning properly is to consume the correct kind of fuel for it. Eating right is still the best way to take care of the body in the long run. But how can you know what the right fuel is? This is where nutrition comes in.

Nutrition is the branch of science that deals with foods and the relationship to health. It examines how a certain organism uses the food and liquids that it ingests for its normal functions, growth, and maintenance. Nutrition is an extremely broad subject which deals from dealing with deficiencies of certain nutrients or vitamins to complex conditions and diseases like hypertension, diabetes, and heart diseases. In modern times, the science of nutrition also covers the "prevention of disease."

The Composition Of The Body

Before we move into the more specific aspects of nutrition concerning IIFYM, let us first look into what the human body is made up of. The human body is made up of many individual parts. They can be grouped and analyzed in different ways.

The Organ Systems

The body is made up of different organs. These organs are further grouped into systems. These systems provide a vital function for the body. Each system, and each organ, requires certain chemicals for them to function properly. They use these chemicals to perform their function—and maybe even more. For example, your muscles require protein for them to grow, which allows them to become stronger. Here are just some examples of the body's organ systems.

> **Skeletal**: This system provides support for the body. The bones serve as anchor points of the muscles and tendons. They also protect vital organs.

Muscular: The muscles in the muscular system are used to move the body. Making them stronger will make performing specific tasks a lot easier.

Digestive: This system turns we eat into nutrients and chemicals that the body can use. It is essentially a single tube that breaks the food down.

Nervous: This is the control center of the whole body.

The Chemical Composition

Every cell of the body is made up of elements. In fact, everything is made up of elements. So we can organize the body into the elements that make it up.

As the late Carl Sagan famously said, "We're made of star-stuff." The human body is made up of the same elements that make up the universe. But we can break the body down into certain molecules that make up the body. We don't need to list down each element that makes up the body.

As we all know, the human body is mostly water. Water makes up about 65% of the body. Protein takes up 20% and Lipids 12%. The remaining 3% is made up of other molecules like RNA and DNA.

Body Composition In Fitness

As we have seen, the body is made up of different elements, chemicals, and molecules that make cells. These cells, in turn, are grouped into organs; and the organs are further grouped into organ systems.

But in terms of fitness, "Body Composition" means something very different. It does not care about the amount.

Rather, body composition in terms of fitness deals with the ratio of fat, bone, muscle, and water in the body. Determining this ratio determines how lean a person is.

There are various ways to determine the composition of a person's body.

Here are some examples.

Body Density

Determining the density of the body is the most accurate way to determine body composition. To calculate the density of anything, you just have to divide its mass by its volume. That is easy for things that have regular shapes made up of a single material or both. But the body does not have a regular shape. And as we said before, it is made up of many different parts.

To determine the density this equation is used:

$$\frac{1}{Db} = \frac{w}{Dw} + \frac{f}{Df} + \frac{p}{Dp} + \frac{m}{Dm}$$

Db = Total Density of the Body

w = Proportion of water

f = Proportion of fat

p = Proportion of protein

m = Proportion of minerals

Dw = Density of water

Df = Density of fat

Dp = Density of protein

Dm = Density of mineral
To calculate the density of the body, just divide the mass by the volume. Weigh the person on a scale to determine his mass. Then, to determine his volume, immerse the person in the water and weigh the water that was displaced. To measure the proportions of water, protein, and other minerals, various chemicals, and tests can be performed. Their densities are then measured or estimated. All that data is then fed into an equation. Determining the proportion of fat can be done by tweaking with the equation.

Ultrasound

Ultrasound can be used to measure the thickness of subcutaneous fat. Its best advantage is it can directly measure the thickness of muscles and intramuscular fat.

Skin Fold

The skin fold test can measure body composition with a caliper. The caliper is used to measure the fat in different places in the body. Once these parts are measured, the total body fat can then be estimated.

ADP

Air Displacement Plethysmography, or ADP, is very similar to water displacement. But instead of using water, the air is used. It uses a special chamber to determine the volume of the body. Then by using the weight or mass of the person, the density can be calculated. The percentage of body fat is then estimated.

DEXA

Dual Energy X-ray Absorptiometry, or DEXA, is said to be the "Gold Standart" in determining the composition of the body. The composition of the body is determined by the machine. It is extremely accurate because it scans the whole body at once. Not only that, but it can also determine other details like bone mineral content, fat tissue mass, and lean tissue mass. This method is performed only by licensed radiologists using the DEXA machine.

CALORIES AND MACRONUTRIENTS

When talking about dieting, most people are concerned about what they eat. They always talk about carbs, fats, and calories. But not everyone understands or even knows what they are. In this section, we will be looking into what calories and macronutrients are.

Calories

When thinking about food intake, people often worry about the calories. They talk about calories as a physical thing. But nobody can show you an example of a calorie. They talk about how much calories a piece of food has, but not the actual calorie itself.

What Are Calories?

Before any diet can be started, you first have to know what the calorie is. The calorie is not a physical thing. You may mistake it for a physical object or thing because of the way people talk about them. You can imagine that each piece of food has little bits of calories within them. But this idea is wrong. A calorie is not a physical thing. It is a unit of measurement.

To define the term "calorie," we have to talk about units of measurement. We all know certain units of measurement like meters, inches, pounds, or ounces. But not everyone knows what the calorie is. But just like any other unit of measurement, the calorie has a scientific definition. A calorie (cal) is "the amount of heat required to raise the temperature of 1 gram of water by 1 degree Celcius." With this definition, you can determine what a calorie is. Again, it is not a physical thing. And, unlike other units of measurement like the meter or the kilogram, there is no physical object to show what it looks like.

But that definition of the calorie is used only is scientific measurements. In terms of food, a different definition is used. The term used in nutrition is called "food calories." It is still connected with the "scientific" calorie. The "calorie" that nutritionists use is the large calorie. The large calorie is the kilocalorie or a thousand "scientific" calories. This is the calorie that we will be more focused on. This is because the "scientific calorie" is just too small. So, when we say "calorie" moving forward, we are talking about the Food Calorie.

Calories and Weight Gain

Now that we have defined the calorie let us now look into its effects on the body. As we said, they are not physical objects. But they affect the body.

Every single piece of food contains calories. The body needs calories to function. It is the fuel that powers the body. However, if the intake of calories exceeds the needs of the body, the exceeding amount is stored as body fat. Not all body fat is bad, because the body needs to have some reserve of energy to use in case of emergency. But having too much fat can be the cause of health issues.

For you not to exceed the required amount, you will need to understand your own caloric needs. Your caloric need is the number of calories that are needed by your body to perform basic functions and your daily activities. In short, your caloric needs will depend on many factors. Metabolism and daily activity are just a couple of them. Caloric needs are also affected by your gender because, generally speaking, men are larger than women, so they require more food. Caloric needs are specific for each individual, but generalizations can be made. The average daily caloric intake recommended for adults is 2000 Cal for females and 2800 Cal for males. For you to find the exact amount of calories your body needs, we will be talking about that later. You may also check out online calculators.

Calories in Food

As we have stated in the previous section, all foods contain calories. This is because they "carry" this fuel for the body. But not all foods are equal. Some contain high calories, while others only have a little. So, let us look into the calorie content of different types and kinds of food.

Beverages

- Beer: 40 kcal

- Coffee: 2 kcal

- Sodas: 40 kcal

- Milo: 425 kcal

- Red Wine: 70 kcal

- White Wine: 65 kcal

Cakes, Deserts, and Sweets

- Cream-filled biscuit: 525 kcal

- White bread (slice): 240 kcal

- Cake: 465 kcal

- Doughnut: 350 kcal

- Custard: 120 kcal

- Pancake: 305 kcal

- Rice: 125 kcal

- Pasta: 115 kcal

Fats and Oils

- Salted butter: 730 kcal

- Margarine: 730 kcal

- Vegetable oils: 900 kcal

Fish and Other Seafood

- Crab: 125 kcal

- Fish fingers: 235 kcal

- Lobster: 120 kcal

- Prawns: 105 kcal

- Tuna: 290 kcal

- Salmon: 155 kcal

Fruits and Vegetables

- Apple: 35 kcal

- Avocado: 225 kcal

- Banana: 80 kcal

- Grapes: 50 kcal

- Grapefruit: 10 kcal

- Mango: 60 kcal

- Orange: 25 kcal

- Peach: 30 kcal

- Pineapple: 45 kcal

- Watermelon: 10 kcal

- Asparagus: 9 kcal

- Cabbage: 25 kcal

- Carrots: 25 kcal

- Celery: 8 kcal

- Cucumber: 10 kcal

- Onions: 25 kcal

- Potato: 85 kcal

- Tomato: 15 kcal

Meat

- Bacon: 475 kcal
- Corned beef: 215 kcal
- Beef fillet steak: 200 kcal
- Chicken leg: 90 kcal
- Chicken wing: 75 kcal
- Hamburger: 225 kcal
- Porkchop: 260 kcal
- Pork sausage: 315 kcal
- Turkey: 170 kcal

As you can see, fruits and vegetables generally contain very low amounts of calories. Oils and meats meanwhile contain quite a lot. But, of course, the calorie content also depends on the serving size. The calorie contents shown here are based on the recommended serving sizes for the foods listed.

Armed with an idea of how many calories each food has, you can make some changes into your food intake in order to lessen the number of calories you ingest. That is basically what dieting is. It is just lowering the number of calories you take in, and sometimes, increasing your physical activities. That is why the IIFYM diet is so much more flexible than other diets. You can skip the exercise part if you don't want to do it. But you will have to lessen your food intake much more. It is best to find a balance between the two in order to gain the best results and keep going for much longer.

Macronutrients

We have discussed the basic ideas and concepts in the science of Nutrition. We have also shown what the body is made up of and how to determine what they are. We have also talked about calories and its effects. Now let us look into the main "course" of this diet: your macros.

What Are Macronutrients?

Macronutrients, or macros, are the main food groups that provide nutrients to your body. They give the most amount of energy in the food you eat. They also serve other functions, but we will look into them into much more detail for each macronutrient.

The three macros are carbohydrates, protein, and fat. Each macro, just like any other food, contains calories as well. But they contain different amounts.

Energy amount per gram:

> **Carbohydrates**: 4 kcal
>
> **Protein**: 4 kcal
>
> **Fat**: 9 kcal

This data is in line with the calorie content we discussed earlier. If you notice, fat contains 9 Calories per gram. That is why, in our list above, the foods with the highest calorie content are fats and oils. Carbohydrates and proteins, on the other hand, contain just 4 calories per gram.

Now, let us look into more detail at each of these macronutrients.

Carbohydrates

Carbohydrates are the most important part of your daily meals. They provide much of the energy that can be used in mental and physical actions. The reason why they are your greatest source of energy is that almost every piece of food has carbohydrates.

Processed foods contain higher carbohydrate levels than unrefined foods. This is because of the process where the shelf life of the product is increased. Many ingredients are added to it that increase its carbohydrate levels.

Carbohydrates come in two major forms: monosaccharides and polysaccharides. The difference comes in their chemical structure.

Monosaccharides are simple carbohydrates and are commonly called sugars. Fructose, or sugar from fruits, and glucose, sugar from starch, are some examples.

Polysaccharides are much more abundant in foods compared to monosaccharides. They are also called complex carbohydrates. They are used by a variety of organisms as energy storage or as structural components. Starch and dietary fiber are some examples.

Sources of Carbohydrates:

- Bananas
- Blueberries
- Rice
- Bread
- Milk
- Potatoes
- Quinoa
- Kidney Beans
- Oats
- Honey

Protein

Protein basically comes from meat. They are made up of long chains of amino acids. The human body cannot synthesize or create protein on its own. That is why you need to add it to your meals.

Protein has many uses in the body, but the main ones are for growth and maintenance. After water, proteins are the most abundant chemical in the human body. It is in all the cells because it is a major component of the cell structure. Proteins, when they are broken down, are also used in cellular repair, hormones, and enzymes. It is also needed in the formation of blood cells.

The intake of proteins is not universal. It depends on a person's physical activity. Physical activities increase the need for protein. Children and breastfeeding women also need to take in protein. The protein in the muscles is also the body's emergency source of energy. This only happens when a person does not eat for several days.

Sources of Protein:

- Meat
- Fish
- Eggs
- Legumes
- Nuts
- Soy Products
- Milk

Fat

Most people are afraid of fat. A lot of diets and eating guides tell you to avoid fats altogether. But what they don't know is that fat carries the flavor in your diet.

Fats, or lipids, can be either solid, like butter, or liquid, like other oils. But they are generally classified into three categories: Saturated Fat, Unsaturated Fat, and Trans Fat.

Unsaturated fats are used by the body to regulate metabolism and to maintain the elasticity of cell membranes. They improve blood flow, and they are also important in the growth of cells and regeneration. They also contain omega-3 and omega-6 fatty acids. These fatty acids are essential for the body, but it cannot synthesize them naturally.

Fats deliver vitamins A, D, E, and K to the body. Animal fats give the body cholesterol, which is used to form vitamin D. Cholesterol is something that most diets say you don't need. But the body does need a bit of cholesterol. Too much of it, though, can increase the risk of cardiovascular diseases.

Sources of Fats:

- **Saturated:** Meat Products, Dairy, Butter

- **Unsaturated:** Olive Oil, Canola Oil, Coldwater Fish, Nuts, Avocados

- **Trans:** Baked Goods, Fried Foods, Margarine

How Important Are Macronutrients?

As we have previously shown, macronutrients come from many kinds of food. We have also touched upon some of their uses. Most diets will tell you to reduce the intake of carbohydrates or fats. Some even tell you to avoid them entirely. But IIFYM does not. Macronutrients are very important and are needed by the body. To be truly healthy, you don't need to give up one of the others. Instead, what you need to strive for is balance.

Foods with carbohydrates are not foods that will make you fat. They are your sources of energy. With enough carbohydrates, you will be able to perform all of your tasks normally and, maybe, with more energy. In a normal diet, carbohydrates should comprise half or 50% of your daily meals.

Proteins are used to treat cells, and the proper amount should be consumed daily. This amount varies from person to person, but it is generally accepted that around 20% of your caloric needs should be protein-rich foods.

Fats generally get a bad "rep" when it comes to diets. This is because most people are trying to get rid of our excess body fats. It is somewhat understandable that they want you to reduce your fat consumption. But not all fats are bad. Unsaturated fats are great for the body. They provide energy and essential fatty acids for the body.

Therefore, it is extremely important that you include all three of these macronutrients in your daily food consumption. You may vary the amounts every single day, even for each meal, but as long as you are getting enough of them, you will be healthy, and you will get that ideal weight. Instead of depriving yourself and your body of the nutrients it needs to strive for balance in all things , make sure that what you eat fits your macros.

CALORIE COUNTING AND MACRONUTRIENT TRACKING

As we have talked about in the previous chapter, calories are units of energy that are used by the body as fuel. We have also discussed what the macros, or macronutrients, are.

Most diets will tell you to reduce the intake of one or more of the macronutrients to lose weight. But removing carbohydrates or fats entirely from your diet may cause health issues instead of helping you out. The best way to reduce weight is by not removing any of the macronutrients from your diet. Instead, it is better just to reduce the number of calories you ingest while still keeping things in balance.

Caloric Needs

Every person needs calories to survive. But not everyone's ideal calorie intake is the same. Multiple factors can change the caloric needs of a specific person.

One of the factors is the amount of physical activity performed by a person. There is going to be a difference between the caloric needs of an athlete and someone who is just sitting all the time. Another factor that can affect the caloric needs of a person is age. Generally speaking, an older person requires fewer calories than a younger person.

For you to reduce weight, there must be a calorie deficit. This is done by taking in fewer calories than you burn off. This, in essence, can be achieved in two ways. One is to increase the number of calories you burn off by exercising more. Another way is to reduce your calorie intake. The better, and probably the faster, way to reduce weight is to combine the two ways: eat less while exercising more.

But you also have to keep in mind that there is a set amount of calories you need every day for you to be still able to do basic things. This is *your* daily caloric need.

As we said before, each person's caloric needs are different. But there is a formula that can help you find what *your* daily caloric needs are. This formula uses a few variables like your age and the amount of physical activity you perform. Plugging the data into the formula will show your daily caloric needs.

Energy Expenditure

Before we get into the equations, we will have to find out how much energy do you use every day. Every activity you perform will consume energy. And, since they are the unit of energy, these actions use calories.

But we first have to find out what the exact number of calories your body needs for every action you perform. Again, this will vary every day, so it will not be exact. What it is is the *average* recommended caloric intake based on the amount of physical activity you perform.

Basal Metabolic Rate and

Resting Metabolic Rate

Your body performs some activities automatically. These actions are, but not limited to, breathing, pumping blood, and brain functions. And, while performing these actions, your body consumes energy. The amount of energy the body requires to keep you alive is your Basal Metabolic Rate or

---

BMR.

There are a lot of calculators online that can help determine your BMR based on several factors. But one of the most common equations that these calculators use is the Mifflin-St Jeor Equation.

$$P = 10(m) + 6.25\left(h\right) - 5(a) + s$$

Where:

P = BMR

m = weight in kilograms

H = height in cm

a = age in years

s = + 5 for males; -161 for females

This equation has been shown to yield the most accurate

results. And with the bonus that it does not require the body fat percentage, which most people do not know.

The Resting Metabolic Rate, or **RMR**, is also another way to measure the body's energy usage when not performing other things. The difference between it and the BMR is that it factors in the energy used when digesting food. The RMR is always higher than BMR because food digestion uses around 10% of a person's energy expenditure.

Total Daily Energy Expenditure

When counting macros, the most important information you can use is your Total Daily Energy Expenditure or **TDEE**. Your TDEE is the representation of all the calories you burn. To lose weight, you need to eat less than your TDEE and not your BMR. Again, just like the BMR, there are a lot of calculators online that can help you calculate your TDEE.

Calculating your TDEE is very simple. You just multiply your BMR to an activity factor. The factors are:

- **Limited Exercise**: 1.2

- **Light exercise**: 1.375

- **Moderate exercise**: 1.55

- **Hard Exercise**: 1.725

- **StrenuousExercise**: 1.9

Once you have determined your TDEE, it is very easy to adjust your diet based on it. You can just eat less than your TDEE to reduce weight or eat more than it to gain weight.

Counting Calories and Macros

We have already shown you how to measure or calculate the number of calories your body needs based on how much physical activity you perform. Let us now look at how you can achieve your goal weight.

These steps will help you get started.

1. Set Your Target

With your TDEE known, you can now set your target. Your target calorie intake will depend on how fast you want to lose weight. On average, decreasing your calorie intake by 20% will yield noticeable results quicker, while still not feeling intimidating. So, if you want to lose weight faster, just decrease your calorie intake even more.

2. Find Your Macro Breakdown

Once you have determined and set your target calorie intake, you can now decide the ratio of macronutrients in your food. The ratio of your macronutrients will help you lose weight even more while still making sure that you are healthy. The Acceptable Macronutrient Distribution Ranges (AMDR) is:

Carbohydrates: 45-65%

Proteins: 10-35%

Fats: 20-35%

This ratio means that, for your daily calorie intake, 45-46% of it should be made up of carbohydrates, and so on. You can still follow other ratios. This is just the recommended ratio.

3. Track your Macros and Calories

To make it easier for you to control how much calories and macronutrients are in your food, it is best to keep a journal where the details of your food are kept. You may also use an app to help you out.

4. Adjust your Intake

There might be times when you underestimate your calorie intake, overestimate the number of calories you expend or both. So it is best to make some adjustments when necessary.

Some Tips for Success

To help you count calories much easier, here are some tips:

- **Prepare**

Prepare all the things or apps you need. It is also best to prepare a meal plan for a week or two.

- **Avoid Junk Food**

Remove all the junk food in your house. Not only will this make sure you don't eat them, but it is also a way for you to look for healthier alternatives.

- **Avoid Processed Food**

Make sure to avoid processed foods. This is for you to get the most nutrients out of the food you are eating. It is best if you make your meals yourself.

- **Read Labels**

Check the labels for all the food. These labels contain a lot of information you can use for calorie counting.

- **Slow and Steady**

Do not aim for immediate or fast weight loss. This will have detrimental effects on your health. And any time when things don't work out, you may give up.

- **Exercise**

All successful techniques for weight loss include not just diet but also exercise. Adjust your diet to compensate for the exercises you perform.

FOOD AND MEAL PLANS

All of your calories and most of your nutrients come from the food you eat. So you must plan the meals you eat.

Planning your meals involves a lot of work and preparation. It can be a bit more complicated when you factor in the calorie and macronutrient contents of the meals you are preparing. Not only will you have to think of what you want to eat, but you will also have to think of what the meal is made up of.

In the previous chapter, we talked about calories and macros. We also talked about the calorie content of each of the macronutrients. The recommended proportions of the macronutrients in your meals have also been discussed. Now, in this section, we will put them all together.

There are some things that you will have to do and things that you have to avoid doing for the IIFYM diet work.

What To Do

For you to be able to create a great meal plan, here are some things that you will have to know to make it work.

Buy in Bulk

One of the biggest considerations when making a meal plan is your budget. Not everyone can dish out lots of money just for food. Most people will have a certain amount of money set for food. So, one of the best ways to follow the IIFYM diet while not breaking the bank is to buy things in bulk.

Buying in bulk not only saves you money, but it will also save you some time. When you have all of your ingredients close at hand, you can easily grab what you need. You won't have to go out and buy that ingredient from the supermarket.

Another time-saving thing that buying in bulk can do is that it helps you plan your meals. This is because you have already set the ingredients you can use. This makes planning what to cook much easier. You just have to look at what you have and prepare your meals.

Prepare Portions

Another way that will help save your time is to prepare all your portions and ingredients beforehand. This will make preparing meals much easier. You can just bring out the ingredients whenever you are ready to cook the meal. You may even cook the meals and then just freeze them. Once you are ready to eat the meal, just reheat it.

Preparing the portions and meals beforehand will not just make cooking a lot easier; it can also help you plan ahead. With the ingredients that you have, you can set what you are going to eat for quite some time, especially if you buy in bulk.

With your meal prepared beforehand, you will not have to worry about tracking your macros and calories every single day. You can plan your intake of macronutrients while preparing the meals and ingredients. This is a great way to save time and to follow the diet with ease.

Keep to your Ratio

We have already calculated the macronutrients and calories that should be in your diet. With the macronutrient ratio and calorie limit you have chosen, you should now be able to determine how much of each macronutrient you should have every day.

As an example, let us calculate how much someone who usually eats 2000 calories per day will need.

First off, to lose weight, the calorie intake should be reduced. The recommended reduction is 20%. So, the calorie intake drops from 2000 kcal to 1600 kcal.

Now, for the percentage of macronutrients. Let us use a 50-20-30 ratio. That is 50% carbohydrates, 20% fat, and 30% protein. Again, this ratio is just an example. Your ratio may be different. You can change things up. However, you want.

So, for this example of 50-20-30, let us calculate the macronutrient calorie counts based on the 1600 kcal diet.

- **Carbohydrates** (50%)

$$1600\frac{kcal}{day} \times .50 = 800kcal$$

$$800kcal \div 4\frac{kcal}{gram} = 200grams$$

Based on this calculation, you should have 200 grams of carbohydrates per day.

- **Fat** (20%)

$$1600\frac{kcal}{day} \times .20 = 320kcal$$

$$320kcal \div 9\frac{kcal}{gram} = 35.5grams$$

Based on this calculation, you should have only 35.5 grams of fats per day.

- **Protein** (30%)

$$1600\frac{kcal}{day} \times .30 = 480kcal$$

$$480kcal \div 4\frac{kcal}{gram} = 120grams$$

Based on this calculation, you should eat 120 grams of proteins per day.

When you have calculated your portions, make sure that you stick to them as much as possible. Track every meal to make sure that you are still within your limit.

Your portions and ratios will differ from other people based on many factors. Some of them may be your gender, age, and amount of physical activity. If you want to lose weight, you may reduce the percentage of carbs and increase the protein.

Use Technology

Nowadays, there are a lot of things that make life a lot easier. There are a lot of apps that can help you track your carbohydrates and macros much easier. There are even apps and websites that give you recipes and ideas on what to make. Websites and apps can even help you save money. There are deals and promotions that you can check out and enjoy.

Buying things online can also make your life easier. You can buy ingredients and spices online on many websites. There are even online services that send prepared ingredients for meals right to your doorstep. They even allow you to customize the meals so that they can fit into your limits. This way, not only are you sticking to the diet, but you are also saving time. Keep in mind, though, that these apps and services may cost more money than if you buy them from a supermarket or grocery store.

You can also use the Internet to search for restaurants that cater to your needs. Whenever you feel like eating out or if you are far from home, you can just go to these restaurants, and you will have a delicious meal that fits your intake.

Experiment

One of the best things about preparing your meals is the cooking process. Even with an old, well-beloved recipe, you can change things up. You can replace some ingredients that will fit your macros and calorie intake.

Trying things out in the kitchen can also lead to some discoveries in food. You never know, on your experimentation, you may even find your new favorite meal. Trying new things out will also allow you to find new ingredients that you may have never used before.

And, just like anything, you should have some "cheat days" where you can eat anything you want. Use these cheat days as a reward for following the diet for some time. You can set your cheat day on any day of the week that you feel. On this day, you can enjoy any kind of food you want.

What To Avoid

On any weight loss program or a healthy diet, there are certain foods that you should not eat. This is a way for you to control your meals and stay healthy. IIFYM is a diet that is much more flexible than others, but as we said before, it is still a diet. There are still some kinds of food that you should avoid. Not only will they break your diet, but some of these foods may even cause illnesses in the long run. There should also be things that you have to remember and follow for you to stick to the diet and still have all the nutrients your body needs.

Lack of Micronutrients

One of the biggest things that the IIFYM diet does not look into is your intake of micronutrients. The IIFYM diet focuses mostly on macros. So, it is up to you to make sure that you are still getting enough micronutrients into your body.

Micronutrients come from a lot of foods. They usually come from fruits and vegetables, but some can also be found in nuts. So when planning or cooking your next meal, make sure to factor in the macronutrients. Your body does not need a lot of them, so you don't have to track how much you are getting. But it is best to find sources for these micronutrients to incorporate them into your meals.

Wrong Kinds of Carbs

Carbohydrates come from a lot of kinds of food. Almost every food you eat will have carbs. But, as we have discussed, there are different kinds of carbohydrates. Complex carbohydrates are the best sources of carbs. The IIFYM diet lets you eat anything, but it is best to keep in mind the *quality* of the food you eat.

Not all carbs are the same. It is not recommended that you eat fast food or processed foods all the time. Not only are they full of carbs that will make you exceed your limit, but they may also have lots of unhealthy fat or oils. Sweet foods should also be limited because of the kind of carbs it contains. Sugary foods usually contain simple carbs instead of complex ones.

When picking your source carbohydrates, make sure to pick the complex ones and keep to your limits.

Ignoring Your Body

Eating based on how much and what a formula tells you to and ignoring what your body tells you can make you miss out on the signals it gives. Your body may be telling you that it needs food, but because of your limits, you are not going to eat. This is wrong. Your calorie intake should be based on how much physical activity you performed for that day. So your meals should adjust accordingly. Not listening to your body may even lead to damage to certain parts of the body.

Whenever you feel hungry, make sure that you eat. You can still follow your percentages but eat what your body tells you to at that moment. You may be lacking certain nutrients, and your body is warning you. Listen to what your body is telling you, and you will stay a lot healthier in the long run. It may mean that you diverge from your daily calorie intake a bit, but at least your body is healthy.

We have talked about what to consider when preparing a meal plan for the IIFYM diet. Let us now look into some examples of recipes that you can follow. Keep in mind that some of these recipes might not fit your calorie limit. These recipes will be 1600 kcal per day or less. So we will be looking at a meal plan with the recipes broken down for every meal. The nutritional information for the recipes is for each serving. Some recipes might have more than one serving.

Day 1

Breakfast

Blueberry and Banana Oats

Ingredients

- Instant steel-cut oats: ½ cup
- Unsweetened vanilla almond milk: ¾ cup
- Banana, sliced: ½
- Blueberries: ½ cup
- Chia seeds: 1 tbsp
- Ground flaxseed: 1 tbsp

Directions

1. Heat up the almond milk.

2. Pour the heated almond milk over the oats.

3. Stir the mixture and let it sit until the oats become thick.

4. Add in the rest of the ingredients.

Nutrition Information:

450 Calories

Fiber: 18 g

Protein: 16 g

Lunch	Ingredients

Avocado BLT

- Whole white bread: 2 slices
- Sliced tomato: 2 pcs
- Banana, sliced: ½

- Turkey Bacon: 3 oz.
- Romaine lettuce leaves: 2 pcs
- Avocado

Directions

1. You may toast the bread if you prefer.

2. Cook the turkey bacon.

3. Spread the avocado on one of the slices of bread. Put the turkey bacon, lettuce, and tomato on top.

4. Top with the second slice of bread.

Nutrition Information:

480 Calories

Fiber: 8 g

Protein: 24 g

Dinner

Mac and Cheese

Ingredients

- Whole wheat penne: ¾ cup

- Shredded cheese (low fat): ½ cup

- Greek yogurt (plain, non-fat): ½ cup

- Garlic powder: 1 tsp

- Spinach: ½ cup

Directions

1. Cook pasta.

2. In an oven dish, mix the pasta, cheese, yogurt, spinach, and garlic powder.

3. Bake until the cheese is crispy on top.

Nutrition Information:

490 Calories

Fiber: 8 g

Protein: 37g

Snack

<u>Trail Mix</u>

Ingredients

- Slivered almonds: 1 tbsp

- Pistachios: 1 tbsp

- Raisins: 1 tbsp

Directions

Mix all ingredients in a bowl.

Nutrition Information:

110 Calories   Fiber: 2 g

Protein: 3 g

Dessert

Frozen Greek Yogurt

Ingredients
- Greek Yogurt: ½ cup

- Raspberries: ½ cup

- Honey: 1 tbsp

Directions

1. Blend all ingredients until smooth.

2. Freeze for about an hour.

Nutrition Information:

70 Calories   Fiber: 4 g

Protein: 13 g

Total Calories: *1 600 Calories*

Day 2

Breakfast

Breakfast Burrito

Ingredients

- Tortilla wrap (wholemeal, warmed): 1
- Egg: 1
- Avocado (sliced): ½
- Cherry tomatoes (halved): 7
- Kale: 50 g
- Chipotle paste: 1 tsp
- Rapeseed oil: 1 tsp

Directions

1. In a jug, mix the chipotle paste and the egg.

2. In a large pan, heat up the oil.

3. Cook the kale and tomatoes in the oil. Push them to the side of the pan once they are cooked.

4. Pour in the egg and chipotle mixture on the clear side of the pan. Scramble all of them together.

5. Put everything in the wrap, and then top with avocado.

Nutrition Information:

366 Calories   Protein: 16 g

Carbohydrates: 26 g

Fat: 21 g

Lunch

Creamy Chicken Quesadillas

Ingredients

- Olive oil: 1 tbsp

- All-purpose flour: 4 tsp

- Chicken stock (unsalted): ½ cup

- Spinach (coarsely chopped) : 1 cup

- Hot sauce: 1 tbsp

- Kosher salt: ¼ tsp

- Black pepper: ¼ tsp

- Boneless rotisserie chicken breast (skinless): 6 oz.

- Mozzarella cheese (preshredded) : 4 oz.

- Whole-wheat flour tortillas (8-in.): 4 pcs

- Cooking spray

- Ripe avocado (quartered)

Directions

1. Cook flour in oil for 30 seconds. Stir constantly.

2. Add the stock slowly and cook it until it thickens.

3. Remove pan from heat.

4. Mix in hot sauce, salt, pepper, cheese, spinach, and cheese.

5. Over medium heat, put a large skillet.

6. Put the chicken mixture on one half of each tortilla. Fold over the filling.

7. Coat quesadillas with cooking spray. Cook on the skillet for 2 minutes each side or until the cheese is melted.

8. Cut into 4 wedges and serve with avocado.

Nutrition Information:

343 Calories   Protein: 23 g

Carbohydrates: 24 g

Fat: 17 g
Dinner

Wild Salmon Vegetable Bowl

Ingredients
- Carrots: 2 pcs.
- Large courgette: 1 pc.
- Beetroot (cooked, diced): 2 pcs.
- Balsamic vinegar: 2 tbsp

- Dill (chopped): ⅓ small pack

- Small red onion (finely chopped): 1 pc.

- Poached or canned wild salmon: 280 g

- Capers in vinegar (rinsed): 2 tbsp

Directions

1. With a peeler or spiralizer, shred the carrots and courgette into long strips.

2. In a small bowl, mix the chopped dill, red onion, beetroot, and balsamic vinegar.

3. Spoon the mixture on the vegetable strips.

4. Flake chunks of salmon.

5. Scatter the salmon flakes and capers on top of the mix. You may add extra dill on top.

Nutrition Information:

395 Calories

Protein: 39 g

Carbohydrates: 18 g

Fat: 17 g

Snack

Baked Pita Chips

Ingredients

- 6-inch Pitas: 4 pcs.
- Olive oil: 2 tbsp.
- Ground cumin: 1 tsp.
- Ancho chile powder: 1 tsp.
- Kosher salt: ¼ tsp.

Directions

1. Preheat the oven to 350°F

2. Cut pitas into 6 wedges. Put them in a large bowl and coat them with oil.

3. In a bowl, mix the salt, chili powder, and cumin. Sprinkle the mixture over the wedges.

4. Place the wedges on baking sheets.

5. Bake them for 12 minutes and let them cool.

Nutrition Information:

148 Calories   Protein: 4.7 g

Carbohydrates: 22.1 g

Fat: 4.6 g

Dessert

Dark Chocolate and Oat Clusters

Ingredients

- Peanut butter: 2 tbsp

- 1% Low-fat milk: 2 tbsp

- Chocolate chips (semisweet): ¼ cup

- Old-fashioned rolled oats: ¾ cup

Directions

1. Mix the milk, peanut butter, and chocolate chips.

2. Heat the mixture in a saucepan over low heat for 3 minutes.

3. Put in the oats. Then remove from heat.

4. Scoop ball-shaped portions on a baking sheet lined with wax paper.

5. Put it in the fridge for 10 minutes.

Nutrition Information:

160 Calories   Carbohydrates: 19 g

Fat: 8 g

Protein: 5 g

Total Calories: 1 412 Calories

Day 3

Breakfast

American Pancakes

Ingredients

- Self-rising flour: 200g
- Baking powder: 1 ½ tsp
- Golden caster sugar: 1 tbsp
- Eggs: 3 pcs
- Butter (melted): 25 g

- Milk: 200ml
- Vegetable oil (for cooking)
- Maple syrup
- Toppings of your choice

Directions

1. In a large bowl, mix the flour, caster sugar, and baking powder. Add in a pinch of salt.

2. Make a small indent in the middle of the mixture.

3. Put the milk, melted butter, and eggs into this indent. Whisk the batter until smooth.

4. Heat a teaspoon of oil and a bit of butter in a large non-stick pan.

5. Pour a bit of batter in the pan. Cook each side for 1-2 minutes.

6. Continue doing this until all the batter is used.

7. Put them on a plate and then pour maple syrup on top. Put in your toppings.

Nutrition Information

356 Calories   Protein: 13 g

Carbohydrates: 46 g

Fat: 13 g

Lunch

Prosciutto, Lettuce, and Tomato Sandwiches

Ingredients

- 100% whole-grain bread: 8 slices

- Canola mayonnaise: ¼ cup

- Fresh basil (chopped): 2 tbsp

- Dijon mustard: 1 tsp

- Small garlic clove (minced): 1 pc.

- Baby romaine lettuce leaves: 1 cup

- Tomato slices (1/4 inch thick: 8 pcs

- Prosciutto (very thin slices): 3 oz

Directions

1. Put bread on a baking sheet. Broil for 2 minutes each side.

2. In a bowl, mix mustard, mayonnaise, basil, and garlic.

3. Spread this mixture on 4 slices of bread.

4. Put a quarter of lettuce on top of each slice of bread. Then 2 slices of tomato. Put prosciutto on top then the other slice of bread.

Nutrition Information

243 Calories   Protein: 11.8 g

Carbohydrates: 28.4 g

Fat: 9.4 g

Dinner

<u>Turkey Burger</u>

Ingredients

- Ground turkey: 1 ½ lb.

- Whole-wheat hamburger buns (1.6-ounce): 6 pcs.

- Granny Smith apple (finely chopped, peeled): $1\frac{1}{3}$ cups

- Greek yogurt (plain, 2% reduced-fat): ½ cup

- Lemon: 1 pc

- Large egg white: 1 pc

- Baby spinach (fresh): 1 ½ cups

- Hot pepper sauce (optional): 1 tsp

- Mango chutney: 2 tbsp

- Salt: 1 tsp

- Freshly ground black pepper: 1 tsp

- Onion (finely chopped): ¼ cup

- Celery (finely chopped): 1 cup

- Cooking spray
- Canola oil: 2 tsp

Directions

1. Heat the canola oil in a large, non-stick skillet on medium-high heat.

2. Saute the celery, onion, and apples for 5 minutes. Set them aside to cool.

3. Grate lemon to get 2 tsp of the rind. Then squeeze to get 1 tbsp of juice.

4. Mix the lemon juice, lemon rind, ground turkey, and the apple mixture in a bowl — season with salt and pepper.

5. Mix in the egg. You may add hot pepper sauce if you prefer.

6. Make 6 patties with a thickness of ½ inch. Put them in the fridge for 2 hours.

7. Preheat the grill and cook the patties for 5 minutes per side.

8. Grill the buns with the cut side down.

9. In a small bowl, mix the yogurt and mango chutney.

10. Assemble the burger. Put patties on the bottom half of the bun, then spinach, pour the sauce.

Nutrition Information

341 Calories per Burger

Fat: 11.2 g

Protein: 28.6 g

Carbohydrates: 33.8 g

Snack

Raspberries with Chocolate Yogurt Mousse

Ingredients

- Greek yogurt (plain, low fat) : ½ cup
- Honey: 1 tbsp
- Raspberries: ¼ cup
- Unsweetened cocoa: 1 tsbp

Directions

1. Mix the honey, yogurt, and cocoa in a small bowl.

2. Put raspberries on top.

NutritionInformation

170 Calories

Protein: 11 g

Carbohydrates: 29 g

Fat: 3 g

Dessert

Fudgy Pudding Pops

Ingredients

- Chocolate almond milk (unsweetened): 2 ½ cups

- Coconut sugar: 1/2 cup

- Unsweetened cocoa: 2 tbsp

- Cornstarch: 1 tbsp

- Bittersweet chocolate (finely chopped): 4 oz.

- Ripe avocado (peeled and pitted): 1 pc

- Vanilla extract: ½ tsp

- Dash of salt

Directions

1. Mix the cocoa, milk, sugar, and cornstarch in a pan.

2. Boil the mix while whisking continuously.

3. Cook the mixture until it thickens.

4. Remove from heat.

5. Add in chocolate. Whisk it until it melts.

6. Let the mixture cool by placing the pan in the bowl with ice.

7. Pour the mixture in a blender. Add avocado, salt, and vanilla.

8. Blend until the mixture is smooth.

9. Pour mixture into popsicle molds.

10. Insert popsicle sticks and freeze for 3 hours.

Nutrition Information

149 Calories   Protein: 2 g

Carbohydrates: 22 g

Fat: 9 g

Total Calories: 1259 Calories

Day 4

Breakfast

Healthy Egg & Chips

Ingredients

- Potatoes (diced): 500 g

- Small mushroom: 200g

- Eggs: 4 pcs

- Shallots (sliced): 2 pcs

- Olive oil: 1 tbsp

- Dried crushed oregano: 2 tsp

Directions

1. Preheat the oven to 400 °F

2. In a large roasting pan, put the potatoes and shallots.

3. Then pour the olive oil and oregano. Mix well.

4. Bake for 45 minutes.

5. Put in the mushrooms and bake for 10 more minutes.

6. Create four spaces in the vegetable mixture.

7. Crack one egg for each space — Bake for 4 minutes.

Nutrition Information

218 Calories   Protein: 11 g

Carbohydrates: 22 g

Fat: 10 g

Lunch

Chicken, Carrot, and Cucumber Salad

Ingredients

- Cooked chicken breast (chopped): 1 lb.

- Cucumber (chopped and seeded): 1 ¼ cups

- Carrots (matchstick-cut) : ½ cup

- Radishes (sliced): ½ cup

- Green onions (chopped): 1/3 cup

- Light mayonnaise: ¼ cup

- Fresh cilantro (chopped): 2 tbsp

- Minced garlic (bottled): 1 tsp

- Salt: ¼ tsp

- Cumin (ground): ¼ tsp

- Black pepper: 1/8 tsp

- Green leaf lettuce: 4 leaves

- 6-inch Whole wheat pitas (cut into 8 wedges): 4 pcs

Directions

1. In a large bowl, combine the chicken, cucumber, carrots, radishes, and chopped green onions.

2. In another bowl, mix the mayonnaise, cilantro, garlic, salt, cumin, and black pepper.

3. Mix the two mixtures and combine them well.

4. On a plate, put one lettuce leaf. Prepare four of these.

5. Put about a cup of the chicken mixture on each leaf.

6. Put 8 pita wedges on top of each plate.

Nutrition Information

382 Calories   Protein: 40.7 g

Carbohydrates: 31.4 g

Fat: 10.4 g

Dinner

<u>Carrot-Ginger Soup</u>

Ingredients

- Butter (unsalted): 3 tbsp
- Olive oil: 3 tbsp

- Onion (chopped): 1 cup

- Fresh ginger (peeled and finely chopped): 2 tbsp

- Garlic (finely minced): 2 cloves

- Chicken or vegetable broth (fat-free, lower-sodium): 7 cups

- Carrot (diced): 4 cups

- Dry white wine: 1 cup

- Fresh lime juice: 2 tsp

- Curry powder: ¼ tsp

- Black pepper (ground): ¼ tsp

- Fresh cilantro (chopped): 2 tsp

Directions

1. Put the butter and olive oil in a large saucepan on medium heat. Cook for 2 minutes, or until the butter melts.

2. Put in the onion, garlic, and ginger. Cook for 10 minutes.

3. Add in the broth, wine, and carrot. Boil and then let it simmer for 45 minutes.

4. Blend the mixture until it is smooth. Make sure to take extra precautions when blending the hot soup.

5. Pour the blended mixture in a bowl. Add in the lime juice, pepper, and curry powder. Stir well.

6. Sprinkle cilantro on top.

Nutrition Information

88 Calories	Fat: 6.4 g
Carbohydrates: 6 g	Protein: 1.2 g

Snack

Zucchini Oven Chips

Ingredients

- Dry breadcrumbs: ¼ cup

- Parmesan cheese (grated): ¼ cup

- Seasoned salt: ¼ tsp

- Garlic powder: ¼ tsp

- Ground black pepper: 1/8 tsp

- Milk (fat-free): 2 tbsp

- Zucchini (¼-inch-thick slices): 2 ½ cups

Directions

1. In a bowl, mix the breadcrumbs, Parmesan cheese, salt, garlic powder, and pepper.

2. In a shallow bowl, pour the milk.

3. Dip a zucchini slice in the milk then coat it with the breadcrumb mix. Repeat for each zucchini slice.

4. Place the slices on an oven rack — Bake at 425 °F for 30 minutes.

Nutrition Information

61 Calories   Protein: 3.8 g

Carbohydrates: 7.6 g

Fat: 1.9 g

Dessert

Dark Chocolate Frozen Banana Bites

Ingredients

- Bananas (cut into 6 slices): 3 pcs

- Cocktail picks: 18 pcs

- Dark chocolate (finely chopped): 5 oz.

- Coconut oil: 2 tsp

- Dried coconut (unsweetened, shredded, toasted): 2 tbsp

- Toasted almonds (chopped): 2 tsp

- Sea salt flakes: ½ tsp

Directions

1. Stick a cocktail pick on each slice of the banana. Place them on a baking sheet. Freeze them for 1 hour.

2. Melt chocolate with olive oil in a double boiler set. Cook for 4 minutes.

3. Dip a skewered banana slice into the melted chocolate.

4. Sprinkle with either coconut, almonds, or salt flakes.

5. Freeze for 1 hour.

Nutrition Information

229 Calories   Protein: 3 g

Carbohydrates: 25 g

Fat: 14 g

Total Calories: 978 Calories

Day 5

Breakfast

Oven-Baked Egg & Chips

Ingredients

- Baking potatoes (cut into wedges): 2 pcs
- Olive oil: 2 tbsp
- Smoked paprika: 1 tsp
- Tomatoes (halved): 2 pcs
- Eggs: 2 pcs

Directions

1. Preheat the oven to 375 °F.

2. Put the potatoes in a roasting tin.

3. Sprinkle paprika and oil on the potatoes. Season with salt and pepper. Mix them well.

4. Roast them in the oven for 25 minutes.

5. Put tomatoes with the cut side up with the potatoes.

6. Create 2 spaces and crack an egg — Bake for 8 more minutes.

Nutrition Information

303 Calories   Protein: 11 g

Carbohydrates: 25 g

Fat: 19 g

Lunch

<u>Creamy Tomato Risotto</u>

Ingredients

- Chopped tomato: 400g can

- Vegetable stock: 1 L

- A knob of butter

- Olive oil: 1 tbsp

- Onion (finely chopped): 1 pc

- Garlic (finely chopped): 2 cloves

- Rosemary (finely chopped): 1 sprig

- Risotto rice: 250g

- Cherry tomato (halved): 300g

- Basil (roughly torn): small pack

- Parmesan (grated): 4 tbsp

Directions

1. Pulse the chopped tomatoes and half of the stock in a food processor until the mixture is smooth.

2. Pour the rest of the stock and the mixture into a saucepan. Let it simmer.

3. In another saucepan, melt the butter with olive oil.

4. Add the onion and cook it for 8 minutes. Put in the garlic and rosemary. Cook for another minute. Add in the rice. Keep stirring for 1 minute.

5. Pour about a quarter of the stock mixture on the rice. Let the rice absorb the stock and then add some more.

6. Once you have poured in about half the stock, put the tomatoes in. Let it cook for 25 minutes.

7. Cover for 1 minute then add the basil. Sprinkle parmesan and black pepper.

Nutrition Information

381 Calories   Protein: 13 g

Carbohydrates: 61 g

Fat: 10 g

Dinner

Spinach and Feta–Stuffed Chicken

Ingredients

- Butter: 1 tbsp
- Garlic (minced): 1 clove
- Baby spinach leaves: 6 cups
- Salt: 1/8 tsp
- Ground black pepper: 1/8 tsp
- Chicken breast halves (skinless, boneless): 4 pcs
- Feta cheese (crumbled): 2 oz.
- Grape tomatoes: 2 cups
- Parmesan cheese: 2 tbsp
- Dry white wine: ¼ cup

Directions

1. Melt the butter in a large skillet. Add the garlic in and cook for 30 seconds.

2. Add baby spinach gradually. Season with salt and pepper. Cook for 2 minutes then remove from heat.

3. Pound the chicken breasts to a thickness of ½ inch.

4. Put feta cheese and spinach on the chicken breasts.

5. Roll the chicken up and secure them with toothpicks.

6. Cook the chicken in the skillet of 3 minutes per side.

7. Add tomatoes then sprinkle Parmesan cheese.

8. Bake for 25 minutes at 425 °F for 25 minutes. Remove chicken from skillet.

9. Pour wine into the skillet to loosen the residue.

10. Cut the chicken into slices.

11. Serve with the tomatoes and the juices from the pan.

Nutrition Information

299 Calories   Protein: 43.7 g

Carbohydrates: 8.1 g

Fat: 8.7 g

Snack

Kale Chips

Ingredients

- Curly kale (trimmed, torn into 2-inch strips): 10½ oz.

- Olive oil: 1 tbsp

- Kosher salt: ¼ tsp

Directions

1. Wash and pat dry the kale.

2. Put them in a large bowl. Drizzle them with olive oil and salt. Toss to mix.

3. Place a single layer of kale in a baking sheet.

4. Bake at 350 °F for 15 minutes.

5. Let them cool and store.

Nutrition Information

67 Calories   Protein: 2.5 g

Carbohydrates: 7.5 g

Fat: 4 g

Dessert

Nectarine-Blueberry Frozen Yogurt Pie Bites

Ingredients

- Dates (pitted): 2/3 cup
- Almonds (toasted): 2/3 cup
- Almond butter: 2 tbsp
- Blueberries: 1/3 cup
- Nectarine (ripe): 1pc
- Plain whole-milk yogurt: ½ cup
- Honey: 1 tbsp

Directions

1. Put the almonds, dates, and almond butter in a food processor and blend them until they are combined.

2. Prepare a muffin pan, and pour the date mixture in the pan. Form little cups.

3. Set aside 12 blueberries and 12 slices of nectarine. Refrigerate them.

4. Mash the rest of the blueberries in a bowl.

5. Finely chop the remaining nectarine. Add them to the mashed blueberries.

6. Add the yogurt and honey to the blueberry mixture. Stir them to combine evenly.

7. Put the mixture in the muffin cups then freeze them for two hours.

8. Before serving, let them stand for about ten minutes and then add a blueberry and nectarine slice on top.

Nutrition Information

216 Calories   Protein: 6 g

Carbohydrates: 26 g

Fat: 12 g

Total Calories: 1 266 Calories

Day 6

Breakfast

<u>Cocoa & Cherry Oat Bake</u>

Ingredients

- Cherries (dried): 75 g
- Chia seeds: 1 tbsp
- Hazelnut milk: 500 ml
- Jumbo porridge oats: 200g
- Cocoa powder: 3 tbsp
- Cocoa nibs: 1 tbsp
- Baking powder: 1 tsp
- Vanilla extract: 1 tsp
- Hazelnuts (blanched): 50 g

Directions

1. Preheat the oven to 395 °F.

2. Put the cherries in a bowl. Pour boiling water over the cherries and set them aside.

3. Soak the chia seeds in 3 tbsp of warm water.

4. Drain the cherries and mix them with the soaked chia seeds.

5. In a large bowl, combine the cherries and chia seeds with the oats, cocoa powder, milk, cocoa nibs, baking powder, and vanilla extract.

6. Put the mixture in an ovenproof dish.

7. Put hazelnuts on top of the mixture then bake for 30 minutes.

8. You may serve this with yogurt and cherry compote.

Nutrition Information

289 Calories   Protein: 9 g

Carbohydrates: 30 g

Fat: 13 g

Lunch

<u>Greek-style roast fish</u>

Ingredients

- Potatoes (wedges): 400g
- Onion (sliced): 1 pc

- Garlic (chopped roughly): 2 cloves

- Oregano (dried or fresh): ½ tbsp

- Olive oil: 2 tbsp

- Lemon (wedges): ½ piece

- Tomatoes (wedges): 2 pcs

- Pollock (skinless fillets): 200 g

- Parsley (roughly chopped): a small handful

Directions

1. Preheat oven to 395 °F.

2. Put the potatoes, garlic, oregano, onion, and olive oil into a roasting tin. Season them with salt and pepper. Mix it well.

3. Roast them for 15 minutes and then turn them over. Bake for 15 minutes more.

4. Put in the lemons and tomatoes. Then roast for 10 minutes.

5. Put the fish fillets on top then bake for 10 minutes.

6. Serve with parsley on top.

Nutrition Information

388 Calories   Protein: 23 g

Carbohydrates. 42 g

Fat: 13 g

Dinner

Parmesan-Crusted Tilapia

Ingredients

- Japanese breadcrumbs (panko) : ½ cup
- Parmesan cheese (grated): 2 oz.
- Kosher salt: ¼ tsp
- Black pepper (ground): ¼ teaspoon
- Eggs (beaten): 2 pcs
- Tilapia fillets (6-ounce): 4 pcs
- Canola oil: 2 tbsp
- Lemon wedges: 8 pcs

Directions

1. In a shallow dish, mix the breadcrumbs, cheese, salt, and pepper.

2. In another dish, put the eggs.

3. Wash the fillets and dry them with paper towels.

4. Dip the fillets into the egg and then into the breadcrumbs.

5. Fry the fish fillets on a skillet with the canola oil. Cook them for 3 minutes per side.

6. Serve with the lemon wedges.

Nutrition Information

305 Calories   Protein: 39.5 g

Carbohydrates: 5.6 g

Fat: 13.6 g

Snack

Fruit Leather

Ingredients

- Sugar: 1 cup

- Lemon juice: ¼ cup

- Apples (peeled, chopped): 4 cups

- Pears (peeled, chopped): 4 cups

Directions

1. Preheat the oven to 150 °F.

2. Line a baking sheet with parchment paper.

3. Blend the sugar, lemon juice, apples, and pears until the puree is smooth.

4. Spread the puree on the pan.

5. Bake in the oven for 6 hours with the oven door slightly open.

6. Once cooked and cooled, tear it up and roll it up for storage.

Nutrition Information

90 Calories   Protein: 0.3 g

Carbohydrates: 23.5 g

Fat: 0.1 g

Dessert

Red Hot Applesauce Gelatin

Ingredients

- Candies (cinnamon red hot): ½ cup
- Water: 1 cup
- Gelatin (cherry-flavored): 1 package (3 ounces)
- Applesauce: 2 cups

Directions

1. Put the water into a saucepan on medium heat.

2. Dissolve the candy in the water.

3. Mix in the gelatin and dissolve.

4. Remove heat and then add the applesauce.

5. Pour into a mold and refrigerate for about 2 hours.

Nutrition Information

78 Calories   Protein: 0.7 g

Carbohydrates: 19.4 g

Fat: 0 g

Total Calories: 1 150

Calories

Day 7

Breakfast

<u>Banana & Tahini Porridge</u>

Ingredients

- Tahini: 1 tbsp
- Milk: 150ml
- Porridge oats: 100g
- Bananas (sliced) : 2 pcs

- Cardamom seeds (crushed): 2 pods
- Sesame seeds (toasted): 1 tbsp

Directions

1. Combine the tahini with 1 tbsp of milk and 1 tbsp of water.

2. In a pan, put in the oats, one of the sliced bananas, the cardamom seeds, 100 ml of milk, and 300 ml of water. Add a bit of salt for taste. Cook them for 5 minutes.

3. Pour the cooked oats into two bowls.

4. Pour the rest of the milk and the other sliced banana on top.

5. Add the tahini mixture on top and sprinkle the toasted sesame seeds.

Nutrition Information

431 Calories   Protein: 14 g

Carbohydrates: 53 g

Fat: 17 g

Lunch

Chinese Pork Chops

Ingredients

- Soy sauce: ½ cup
- Brown sugar: ¼ cup
- Lemon juice: 2 tbsp
- Vegetable oil: 1 tbsp
- Ground ginger: ½ tsp
- Garlic powder: 1/8 tsp
- Pork chops (boneless): 6 pcs

Directions

1. Combine all the ingredients except the pork chops in a bowl. Set a little bit of the mixture as a marinade.

2. With a fork, pierce the sides of the porkchop. Place them in a container and pour the marinade in. Refrigerate the pork chops for 8 hours.

3. Preheat the grill.

4. Cook the pork on the grill for about 8 minutes for each side.

5. Brush the pork with the little bit of the marinade you set aside while cooking.

Nutrition Information

182 Calories   Protein: 19.6 g

Carbohydrates: 11.2 g

Fat: 6.3 g

Dinner

<u>Sesame Ramen</u>

Ingredients

- Instant noodles: 80g pack

- Spring onions (finely chopped): 2 pcs

- Pak choi: ½ head

- Egg: 1 pc

- Sesame seeds: 1 tsp

- Chilli sauce (for serving)

Directions

1. Cook the instant noodles by following the instructions on the pack.

2. Add the pak choi and spring onions once the noodles are cooked.

3. Boil the egg.

4. In a frying pan, toast the sesame seeds.

5. Pour the noodles into a bowl.

6. Cut the egg in half and put them on top of the noodles.

7. Sprinkle the sesame seeds on top.

8. You may also put the chili sauce in.

Nutrition Information

205 Calories   Protein: 11 g

Carbohydrates: 21 g

Fat: 7 g

Snack
Fruit Skewers

Ingredients

- Strawberries (halved): 5 pcs

- Cantaloupe (balls or cubes): ¼ piece

- Bananas (chunks): 2 pcs

- Apple (chunks): 1 pc

- 20 skewers

Directions

1. Stick the pieces of fruit onto the skewer. You may vary the order based on what you like.

2. Place them onto a serving platter.

Nutrition Information

61 Calories

Carbohydrates: 0.9 g

Fat: 0.3 g

Protein: 15.4 g

Dessert
Peach Upside-Down Cake

Ingredients

- Peaches: 6 pcs

- White sugar: 2/3 cup

- Butter (unsalted): 2 tbsps

- All-purpose flour: 1 cup

- Baking powder: 1 tsp

- Baking soda: ½ tsp

- Ground cinnamon: ½ tsp

- Salt: ¼ tsp

- Canola oil: 1 tbsp

- Egg: 1 pc

- Vanilla extract: 1 tsp

- Almond extract: 1 tsp

- Low-fat buttermilk: ½ cup

Directions

1. Preheat your oven to 375 °F.

2. Boil the peaches in water until the skins are soft. Peel and halve them and remove the pits.

3. Cook half of the sugar with a tablespoon of butter for 5 minutes.

4. Put the peaches with the cut side up on the sugar. Then remove from heat.

5. In a bowl, mix the flour, baking soda, baking powder, salt, and cinnamon.

6. In another bowl, mix the remaining sugar and butter with the canola oil.

7. Add the egg until the mixture is smooth.

8. Put in the vanilla extract and almond extract.

9. Put the buttermilk and the flour mixture to the sugar. Mix them until the mixture is smooth.

10. Spread the batter on top of the peaches.

11. Put the peaches into the oven and bake for 25 minutes. Let it cool for 5 minutes after it is cooked.

12. Serve by inverting the skillet into a plate. Replace any peaches that stick to the skillet into the cake.

Nutrition Information

137 Calories   Carbohydrates: 23.8 g

Fat: 3.7 g

Protein: 2 g

Total Calories: 1 016 Calories

These recipes are just some examples of what you can eat. As we said earlier, you can switch things up or replace certain meals in the plan we put. If you notice, all the recipes add up to less than 1600 calories per day. Some of them even go much lower. So, if you feel that the number of calories is too low for you, you may look into some foods that can "add up" some more calories.

Another thing that these recipes do not factor in is your physical activity. The recipes do not consider whether you are exercising or not. If you are exercising, the number of calories you have to take in will increase. You may also have to change the ratio of your macros to suit your physical exertions.

What you have to keep in mind is that these recipes only serve as a guide for you to create your meal plan. Make sure that your meals fit your macros, your needs, and, of course, your budget.

TRACKING YOUR PROGRESS

Tracking the kind of food you eat will take a lot of effort and discipline. It is just so easy to give in to temptation and eat whatever you see. That is the underlying beauty of the IIFYM diet. You don't have to worry about what you eat. You just have to consider how much of it you eat and burn off. As long as it fits your macros and caloric needs, you can eat it!

One of the best ways for you to make sure that the food you are eating does fit your macros is to track what you eat. There are several ways you can do this so that we will be looking at some of them.

Journal

Journals are great for tracking your intake of calories and macronutrients. It is very simple to do. You can customize the journal to your liking and make it look good. There are many decorations that you can put in your journal. But keeping it simple will be your best bet.

To do this properly, you will need information from what you eat. It is best to track every meal you eat and then jot the information down into your journal. This is a great way to make sure that you are getting all the information about what you are eating and keeping to the limits you set.

The great thing about the journal is that it allows you to make choices about what you eat. Since you are tracking the macros and not just calories, you will see the difference in the quality of what you are eating.

Tracking Board

A tracking board is extremely similar to your journal—except it is bigger and more conspicuous. It is also a bit more temporary unless you have a big board. A tracking board is a great way to look at your progress at a glance. It is better if you use this with the journal. With your tracking board, you can create graphs or charts to show how much you have progressed. It can also be used as a way to get ideas about what you can eat or more information about the diet.

Apps

In this modern age, there are a lot of great pieces of technology that you can help you out to track your progress and what you eat. Using technology can make things a whole lot easier to follow the IIFYM diet and make sure that you are getting enough macros and calories.

As we briefly said before, there are multiple apps that you can use to help you with the IIFYM diet. There are many similarities between them. Most of them allow you to enter the information about what you are eating and calculate or show the macros and the calories in the meal. Some of them even come with calculators that calculate the macros your need based on your information. Some of them also track the physical activity you perform.

Most of the apps also function as meal planners. These apps provide menus and recipes with all the information you will need to follow the diet. You can even order the ingredients for the meal directly on the app and have them delivered to you!

CONCLUSION

The IIFYM diet is one of the newer dieting regimens that is gaining a bit of traction in recent times. IIFYM is an acronym that means "If It Fits Your Macros." It is a flexible, dieting regime that allows you to eat whatever you want. It works by tracking how much you eat instead of *what* you eat.

The IIFYM diet changes how you think about how the body gets fat. Most people think that certain foods will make you fat. But what they do not realize is that it is the excess of calories that make the body gain weight. So, the IIFYM diet is a way to control the calorie intake of the body.

The IIFYM diet has a lot of benefits, but of course, there are some not so good things about it as well. One of the advantages is that you can, of course, lose weight or at least get the weight you want. It is also very flexible because you can eat whatever you want—as long as it fits your macros. Because of this, there are no "forbidden" foods. This means that you can eat whatever you want. Because it reduces the intake of calories, the IIFYM may require less exercise to achieve results.

One of the main disadvantages of the IIFYM diet is that it is still a diet. This is because most diets are not very sustainable in the long run. So quite a lot of discipline will be required. Also, the IIFYM—as the name suggests—focuses all of its attention on macronutrients but does not care about micronutrients. Micronutrients are very important to the body, and inadequacy of them can result in some illnesses. To overcome this, it is best to incorporate micronutrient supplements into the diet. Another not-so-good thing about the IIFYM diet is that certain health conditions are not accounted for in the calculation of calorie and macronutrient intake. The IIFYM diet, because it is still a diet, can sometimes lead to eating disorders.

The body has been compared to a machine. The food you eat is extremely important because it is the fuel of the body. Nutrition is the branch of science that involves food intake and health. The composition of the body is a very important part of nutrition. The body can be broken down into organ systems or based on the chemical composition.

In fitness, though, body composition means something very different. It pertains to how much muscles, fat, and bone is in the body. The ratio of fat to muscle is often a great indicator of overall health. This can be done through different methods. Calculating the density of the body is one of the most common ways to do it. Various indirect ways of determining body composition are also available. Ultrasound, Skin Fold method, Air Displacement Plethysmography (ADP) are just some examples. But the best one available right now is called the Dual Energy X-ray-Absorptiometry. It is a very accurate way to determine the composition of the human body.

One of the biggest misconceptions about food and nutrition, in general, is about calories. Most people think off calories as some physical object that a piece of food has. But that is not what a calorie is. First and foremost, the calorie is a unit of measurement. It is the most basic unit of measuring energy. It boils down to *"the amount of heat required to raise the temperature of 1 gram of water by 1 degree Celcius."* But that is the scientific definition of the calorie. The Calorie used when nutrition and food is the *kilo*calorie—or a thousand *calories*. This is what causes the body to gain weight. In essence, the more calories you take in, the more weight you gain. But different kinds of food have different calorie contents. To make sure that you are eating right, you have to know how many calories do you need every day.

Macronutrients, sometimes called macros, are in the main kinds of food, or food groups, that provide the most nutrients for the body. They pack a lot of energy and are the main sources of energy that the body uses. The macronutrients are Carbohydrates, Proteins, and Fats.

Carbohydrates, or carbs, contain 4 kcal for every gram. They give a lot of the energy you need every day because they are so abundant. Carbs can be found on pretty much every kind of food you eat. Fruits, vegetables, bread, and dairy products have carbs in them. They often make up half, or 50%, of the food you eat every single day.

Proteins come from meat. The human body cannot create proteins, but it is needed for muscle growth and regeneration. So it should be incorporated into the diet. Proteins can be found in meat, fish, eggs, and some nuts.

Fats are the carriers of flavor in the diet. They contain 9 kcal per gram, so that means you will need less of them in order not to exceed your daily needs. Fats are used by the body to regulate metabolism and for the maintenance of the elasticity in the cell membranes. They also deliver vitamins A, D, E, and K. Fats are used in a lot of foods, but they function as additives or are part of the cooking process.

These three macronutrients—carbs, proteins, and fats—serve extremely important roles in the body. A lot of new diets say that to reduce weight; you have to reduce the intake of one or more of these macros. Some even advise you to remove them from your diet completely. This is the wrong way of losing weight. You are not only depriving your body of essential nutrients, but doing so may even lead to illnesses and nutrient deficiencies.

The body needs calories to function. They are the fuel that makes the bodywork. But not every person requires the same number of calories. Some people need more calories because they are more active. While others may require less because of their age, these are just some of the factors that affect the caloric needs of a person. But the most basic thing you have to understand is that the intake of calories is directly proportional to weight gain. That is the most basic way to put it. The more calories you take in, the more weight you will gain. The more you burn, the more you weight you lose. But you also have to keep in mind that your body requires a certain number of calories to function normally. The body needs them to keep your heart, brain, and other vital organs running. This is called the Basal Metabolic Rate or BMR. It is based on your age, weight, and height. The RMR, or Resting

Metabolic Rate, on the other hand, is a little bit higher than the BMR. This is because it factors in the energy used by digesting the food you eat. So, to calculate the number of calories you require every day based on your physical activity, you will need to calculate your TDEE or Total Daily Energy Expenditure. Once you have that information, you can now calculate how many calories you need to lose weight or gain some.

Counting the calories, you take in seems like a daunting task. It does take a lot of discipline and strength, but it is very simple. You just have to make sure that, whatever you eat, it does not exceed your daily allowance. To do this, you will have to set goals or targets. Once you have done that, it is just a matter of meeting those targets. There are a lot of ways you can do this, but the best and simplest way is just to find a breakdown of macros that fits your needs. Tracking your intake may seem tedious, but it is necessary for you to make sure that you are on track. It is also a great way of motivating you to see how much you have changed. Also, do not forget to adjust or make changes based on specific circumstances.

The best way to make sure that you are keeping within your target is to make a meal plan. Meal plans are charts and recipes that calculate the macros and calories within the meal. They are also time-saving techniques that can make following the diet much easier. Preparing ingredients, or even whole meals beforehand can help you out. Not only will you save time, but you will also be able to calculate your intake much more accurately. To save time and money, buying things in bulk and on sale will help. You can also use apps, websites, and other pieces of technology to make tracking your intake of calories and macros much easier. But most of all, do not forget to experiment from time to time. Enjoy the process, and the results will be worth it. But make sure that you factor in macronutrients into your meals. Look for meals and ingredients that give a better quality of nutrients. Not all sources of macros are the same—so keep that in mind. Most importantly, never ignore the signals that your body is giving. If you are feeling hungry, make sure that you eat even if it means going over your limits.

There are countless recipes that you can follow online. You can incorporate them into your meal plan. Just make sure that they fit within your limit. If you are looking for recipes online, make sure that you get the nutritional information for that meal—especially for the macros.

Tracking your progress with the IIFYM diet is very simple. You just have to take note of what you are eating and log it. But there are multiple ways you can take note of your calorie and macro intake. You can use a journal because it is very simple and easy to use. You may also use a tracking board to have a visual display of your progress. Right now, there are a lot of apps and websites that can help you track and take note of your progress. These apps and web sites can function as a journal because they let you take note of what you are eating. They are also like tracking boards because they show your progress at a glance. But one advantage these apps have over more traditional methods is their connectivity and the number of things you can do with them. Most apps have calculators for all the information you will need, like your BMR and TDEE. Some factors in the amount of exercise that you do. Other apps, meanwhile, contain a whole database of recipes and cooking instructions to help you plan your meals and cook them. You can even shop for supplies and ingredients straight in the app!

No matter what avenue or technique you choose to attain your goal, you have to keep in mind the reason why you are doing this. The IIFYM diet is not just a plan for you to achieve the body that you want. It is part of the diet, but getting the perfect body is not the main goal of the IIFYM diet. The main purpose of the IIFYM diet is for you to be healthy. No matter what shape you are in, you can be healthy. That is the beauty of this diet. It does not dictate what you can or cannot eat—you can eat whatever you want. Just make sure that you are sticking within your target. You are responsible for your health. You are responsible for what kind of fuel you use to power the machine that is your body. For you to be strong and healthy, you should give your body the correct kind of fuel that it needs. Do everything in your power to be healthier, and that ideal body you have been dreaming of will follow.

FINAL WORDS

Thank you again for purchasing this book!

We hope this book can help you.

The next step is for you to **join our email newsletter** to receive updates on any upcoming new book releases or promotions. You can sign-up for free, and as a bonus, you will also receive our "*7 Fitness Mistakes You Don't Know You're Making*" book! This bonus book breaks down many of the most common fitness mistakes and will demystify many of the complexities and science of getting into shape. Having all this fitness knowledge and science organized into an actionable step-by-step book will help you get started in the right direction in your fitness journey! To join our free email newsletter and grab your free book, please visit the link and signup: **www.effingopublishing.com/gift**

Finally, if you enjoyed this book, then we would like to ask you for a favor, would you be kind enough to leave a review for this book? It would be greatly appreciated! Thank you, and good luck with your journey!

ABOUT THE CO-AUTHORS

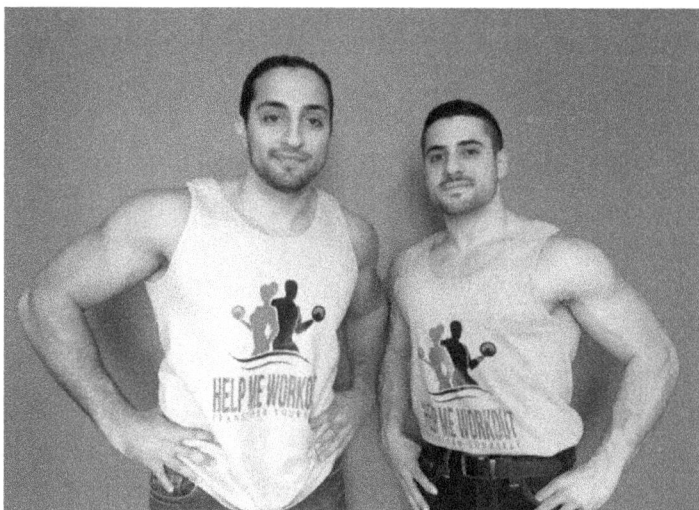

Our name is Alex & George Kaplo; we're both certified personal trainers from Montreal, Canada. We will start by saying we are not the biggest guys you will ever meet, and this has never really been our goal. We started working out to overcome our biggest insecurity when we were younger, which was our self-confidence. You may be going through some challenges right now, or you may simply want to get fit, and we can certainly relate.

We always kind were interested in the health & fitness world and wanted to gain some muscle due to the numerous bullying in our teenage years. We figured we could do something about how our body looks like. This was the beginning of our transformation journey. We had no idea where to start, but we both just got started. We felt worried and afraid at times that other people would make fun of us for doing the exercises the wrong way. We always wished we had a friend to guide us and who could just show us the ropes.

After a lot of work, studying, and countless trials and errors. Some people began to notice how we were both getting more fit and how we were starting to form a keen interest in the topic. This led many friends and new faces to come to us and ask us for fitness advice. At first, it seemed odd when people asked us to help them get in shape. But what kept us going is when they started to see changes in their own body and told us it's the first time that they saw real results! From there, more people kept coming to us, and it made both of us realize after so much reading and studying in this field that it did help us, but it also allowed us to help others. To date, we have coached and trained numerous clients who have achieved some pretty amazing results.

Today, both of us own & operate this publishing business, where we bring passionate and expert authors to write about health and fitness topics. We also run an online fitness business, and we would love to connect with you by inviting you to visit the website on the following page and signing up for our e-mail newsletter (you will even get a free book).

Last but not least, if you are in the position we were once in and you want some guidance, don't hesitate and ask... We will be there to help you out!

Your coaches,

Alex & George Kaplo

Download another book for Free

We want to thank you for purchasing this book and offer you another book (just as long and valuable as this book), "Health & Fitness Mistakes You Don't Know You're Making," completely free.

Visit the link below to signup and receive it:

www.effingopublishing.com/gift

In this book, we will break down the most common health & fitness mistakes, you are probably committing right now, and will reveal how you can easily get in the best shape of your life!

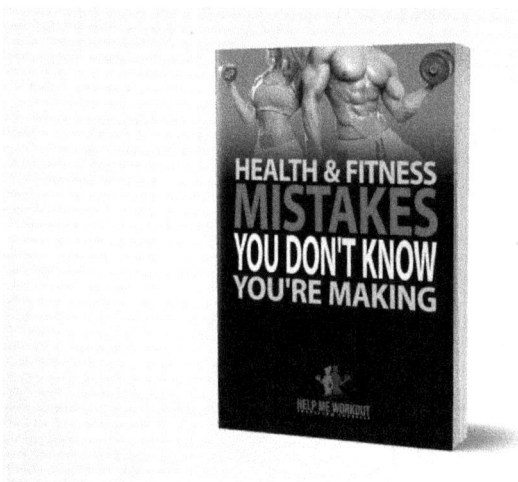

In addition to this valuable gift, you will also have an opportunity to get our new books for free, enter giveaways, and receive other valuable emails from us. Again, visit the link to sign up:

www.effingopublishing.com/gift

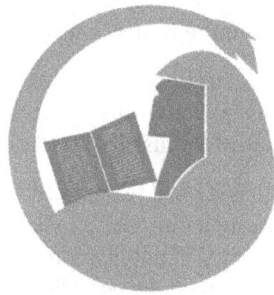

EFFINGO
Publishing

For more great books, visit:

EffingoPublishing.com

www.ingramcontent.com/pod-product-compliance
Lightning Source LLC
Chambersburg PA
CBHW050728030426
42336CB00012B/1469